CW00820662

THE NEW DASH COOKING

A Cookbook That Contains Recipes for Taking the First Step in a More Healthy and Sustainable Lifestyle

Dash and Delicious

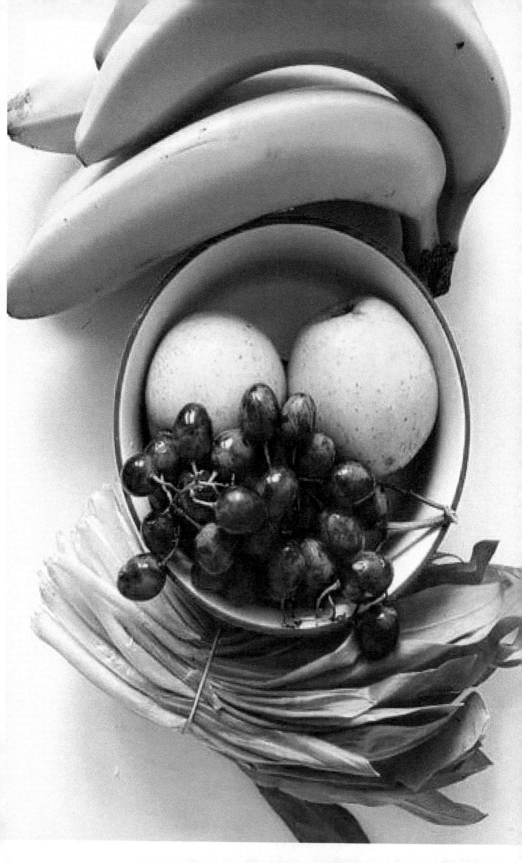

© Copyright 2021 by Dash and Delicious- All rights reserved.

The following Book is reproduced below to provide information that is as accurate and reliable as possible. Regardless, purchasing this Book can be seen as consent to the fact that both the publisher and the author of this book are in no way experts on the topics discussed within and that any recommendations or suggestions that are made herein are for entertainment purposes only. Professionals should be consulted as needed before undertaking any of the actions endorsed herein.

This declaration is deemed fair and valid by both the American Bar Association and the Committee of Publishers Association and is legally binding throughout the United States.

Furthermore, the transmission, duplication, or reproduction of any of the following work including specific information will be considered an illegal act irrespective of if it is done electronically or in print. This extends to creating a secondary or tertiary copy of the work or a recorded copy and is only allowed with the express written consent from the Publisher. All additional rights reserved.

The information in the following pages is broadly considered a truthful and accurate account of facts and as such, any inattention, use, or misuse of the information in question by the reader will render any resulting actions solely under their purview. There are no scenarios in which the publisher or the original author of this work can be in any fashion deemed liable for any hardship or damages that may befall them after undertaking the information described herein.

Additionally, the information in the following pages is intended only for informational purposes and should thus be thought of as universal. As befitting its nature, it is presented without assurance regarding its prolonged validity or interim quality. Trademarks that are mentioned are done without written consent and can in no way be considered an endorsement from the trademark holder.

Table of Contents

INTRODUCTION

The last two decades have witnessed a doubling in the number of people with high blood pressure, many of whom are not good at controlling their symptoms. Our millennial lifestyle has played a great role in producing this worrisome result.

To counter this, scientists introduced the DASH diet, which is an effective way to counteract hypertension among people. The diet is results of careful study of the various food items that will help people control their blood pressure levels.

What is the DASH diet?

Endorsed by the United States National Heart, Lung, and Blood Institute, the DASH (Dietary Approaches to Stop Hypertension) diet studies the nutrient composition of food to prepare unique dietary strategies to eliminate the foods that contribute to high blood pressure.

The United States Department of Health and Human Services began to look for ways to deal with hypertension and eliminate the various risks that are associated with it. Researchers found that people who consume more vegetables or followed a plant-based diet had less of a risk of high blood pressure. This, therefore, became the foundation of the DASH diet.

This diet focuses on foods that are non-processed and more organic. Whole grains, fruits, vegetables, and lean meats form the essential components. In extreme cases, where signs of heart-related ailments due to high blood pressure are present, it is advised for the patient to go vegan for some time to lower issues related to hypertension.

The Dash diet strict dietary sodium because too much salt and oil significantly raise blood pressure. The dietary guidelines of the DASH diet significantly reduce the intake of salt. The recipes in the DASH diet are a wholesome mix of green vegetables, natural fruits, low-fat dairy foods, and lean protein such as chicken, fish, and beans. Besides limiting the intake of salt, the rule of thumb is to minimize food items rich in red meat, processed sugars, and composite fat.

Benefits of the DASH diet

The benefits of the DASH diet go beyond reducing hypertension and heart ailments.

- **Controlling blood pressure**

The force exerted on our blood vessels and organs when the blood passes through them is a measure of blood pressure in the human body. When blood pressure increases beyond a certain level, it can lead to various bodily malfunctions, including heart failure.

Blood pressure is counted in two numbers: systolic pressure and diastolic pressure. Normal blood systolic pressure in adults is below 120 mmHg, while the diastolic pressure is typically below 80 mmHg. Anyone over these limits is said to be suffering from high blood pressure.

The restriction of sodium intake and reliance on vegetables, healthy fat, lean meat, and fruits in the DASH diet greatly controls blood pressure. Effective use of the DASH diet can control the systolic blood pressure by an average change of 12 mmHg and can control the diastolic blood pressure by 5 mmHg.

The DASH diet is not reserved for people suffering from hypertension; it can also work well for people with normal blood pressure. The trick is to consume normal amounts of salt along with the dietary recommendations given in the DASH diet.

- **Weight loss**

People with high blood pressure are advised to maintain an optimal weight, as extra weight may translate into health complications. Obesity along with high blood pressure can lead to heart and organ failure. With the help of the DASH diet, one can lower their blood pressure while also reducing their weight. The credit for this goes to the healthy foods recommended in the DASH diet.

Further, the DASH diet has shown signs of other health benefits:

- **Lowers the risk of cancer**

People on the DASH diets have a lower risk of colorectal and breast cancers.

- **Checks metabolic syndrome**

The diet reduces the risk of metabolic syndrome.

- **Controls diabetes**

The diet is very beneficial for people with type 2 diabetes.

- **Heart diseases**

The diet reduces the risk of heart disease and stroke.

DASH Food Guidelines - What to Eat and Avoid on the Dash Diet

On the DASH diet, excessive fats, salt, and spices need to be avoided. Cut all empty carbohydrates from the diet completely, opting for food that is rich in vitamins, protein, and fiber.

DASH Foods and Serving Sizes

One of the important features of the DASH diet is 'proportion.' Correct proportion of food portions is essential. How do you determine the proportions? Based on extensive research and years of studies, experts have recommendations for serving sizes and combination, depending on nutritional value. The following table shows the serving size of all the major categories of food in a certain caloric diet.

Foods to Enjoy

On a broader scale, this diet plan doesn't restrict the use of most food items, but it does limit their amount. Following is the list of items that can be taken on the DASH Diet:

Seeds	Fruits	Poultry
Nuts	Vegetables	Seafood
Grains	low fat or no-fat dairy products	Beef
		Pork

- **Vegetables: 4-5 Servings Daily**

A half cup of cooked or raw vegetables or 1 cup of leafy vegetables constitutes one serving on the DASH diet. Carrots, greens, sweet potatoes, broccoli, and tomatoes can all be included by adjusting the values of the serving. Set the limiting values and fill in as many vegetables as you can.

- **Grains: 6-8 Servings Daily**

Rice, pasta, cereal, quinoa, bread, etc., are all considered grains. A single serving means 1 oz. of cereal, 1 slice of bread, or a half cup of pasta or rice. Keeping these proportions in mind, you can consume a single serving six to eight times per day. How you divide these servings in a day depends completely on you. Whole grains are recommended most as they are rich in fiber. Similarly, go for brown rice and whole-wheat pasta; both have more fiber.

- **Dairy: 2 - 3 Servings Daily**

Dairy products include cheese, milk, and yogurt. All are a source of protein, calcium, and vitamin D. As long as the dairy products are free from saturated fats or contain a low amount of fat, they are good to go for the DASH diet. A single serving means 1 cup of low-fat yogurt or skim milk or 1.5 oz. of part-skim cheese.

- **Fats and oils: 2 - 3 servings Daily**

Good cholesterol fats and plant-based fats are great for the body; in fact, they strengthen the immune system and aid the absorption of vitamins in the body. Excluding them completely from your diet is unnecessary and unhealthy. Place them in the middle category, having three servings a day, and focus more on mono-saturated fats.

- **Fruits: 4 - 5 Servings Daily**

One medium-sized fresh fruit or canned fruits make a single serving. Fruits are packed with fiber, minerals, and vitamins, so they are good additions to the DASH diet. They generally have low or zero sodium. Four oz. of fruit juice makes up a single serving. Add all the varieties to set the final figures up to five servings in a day.

- **Sweets: 5 servings a week**

Sweets should be consumed least. Five servings a week is more than enough. One serving is one tbsp sugar, a half cup of sorbet, or a cup of lemonade. A moderate use of sweets is necessary; complete deprivation would result in more harm.

- **Seeds, Nuts, and legumes: 4 - 5 Servings Per Week**

This category includes lentils, kidney beans, and peas, edibles seeds like sunflower, sesame, and almonds. They all are a great source of potassium, protein, and magnesium. They are rich in fiber and antioxidants, which prevent cancer and cardiovascular diseases.

Foods to Avoid

Food that can cause hypertension, high blood pressure, high blood sugar levels, and obesity are all forbidden on a DASH diet. The following list of items should be limited:

1. Salt
2. Sugary beverages
3. Processed food
4. High fat dairy products
5. Salted nuts
6. Excessive animal-based fats

Some Questions regarding the DASH DIET

Q. Can people without hypertension also use the DASH diet?

The DASH diet was indeed created to reduce the risk of hypertension and control blood pressure, but owing to its wide-ranging health benefits, anyone can use this diet for better health.

Q. How long should a dieter stick to the DASH diet to see the results?

It is best to make this plan a lifestyle if you are a hypertension patient, rather than adopting it for a few days or months. Since it does not harm you in the long run, it is up to you and your health expert to follow this diet plan as long as needed.

Q. What can you drink on the DASH diet?

All low-calorie, sodium-free, and sugar-free drinks are most suitable for the DASH diet, which make water a perfect candidate. However, sugar-free juices and drinks are also a good option.

Q. Can you use the DASH diet when you are taking medications for hypertension or high blood pressure?

It is not suggested to use the DASH diet when you are on any medication as there can be interactions. Ask for your doctor's opinion on this matter and take his advice to continue the medications along with the diet or not.

BREAKFAST

Cherries Bowls

6 Servings

Preparation Time: 10 minutes

Ingredients

- 4 tablespoons Coconut sugar
- 4 cups non-fat Yogurt
- 1 cup Cherries, pitted and halved
- ½ teaspoon Vanilla extract

Directions

- In a bowl, combine the yogurt with the cherries, sugar and vanilla, toss and keep in the fridge for 10 minutes.
- Divide into bowls and serve f breakfast.

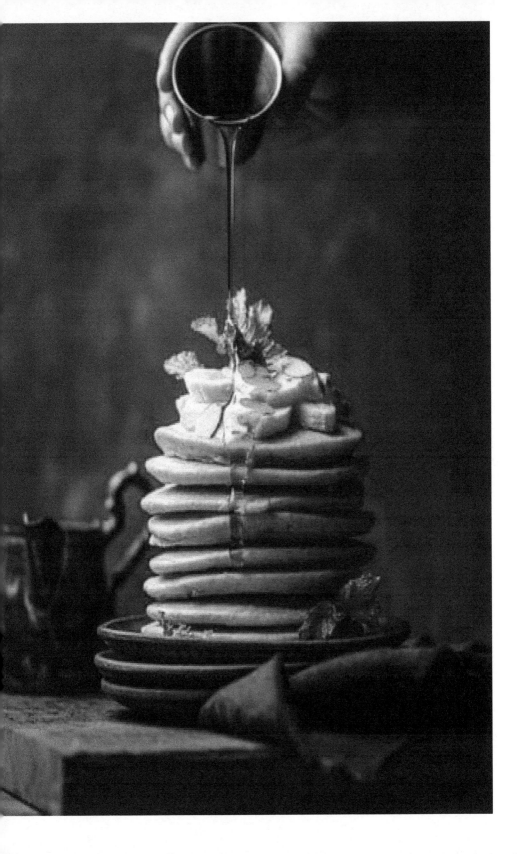

Cinnamon Plums

6 Servings

Preparation Time: 25 minutes

Ingredients

- 1 cup Coconut cream
- 4 Plums, pitted and halved
- 3 tablespoons Coconut oil, melted
- ½ teaspoon Cinnamon powder
- ¼ cup unsweetened Coconut, shredded
- 2 tablespoons Sunflower seeds, toasted

Directions

- In a baking dish, combine the plums with the oil, cinnamon and the other ingredients, introduce in the oven and bake at 380 degrees F for 15 minutes.
- Divide everything into bowls and serve.

Apples Bowls

6 Servings

Preparation Time: 10 minutes

Ingredients

- 2 tablespoons Coconut sugar
- 2 cups non-fat Yogurt
- 6 Apples, cored and pureed
- 1 cup natural Apple juice
- 1 teaspoon Cinnamon powder

Directions

- In a bowl, combine the apples with the apple juice and the other ingredients, stir, divide into bowls and keep in the fridge for 10 minutes before serving.

Strawberry Oats

6 Servings

Preparation Time: 30 minutes

Ingredients

- 2 cups Strawberries, sliced
- 1 and ½ cups Gluten-free oats
- 2 and ¼ cups Almond milk
- ½ teaspoon Vanilla extract
- 2 tablespoons Coconut sugar

Directions

- Put the milk in a pot, bring to a simmer over medium heat, add the oats and the other ingredients, stir, cook for 20 minutes, divide into bowls and serve for breakfast.

Almond Peach Mix

6 Servings

Preparation Time: 25 minutes

Ingredients

- ¼ teaspoon Almond extract
- 6 Peaches, cored and cut into wedges
- ¼ cup Maple syrup
- ½ cup Almond milk

Directions

- Put the almond milk in a pot, bring to a simmer over medium heat, add the peaches and the other ingredients, toss, cook for 15 minutes, divide into bowls and serve for breakfast.

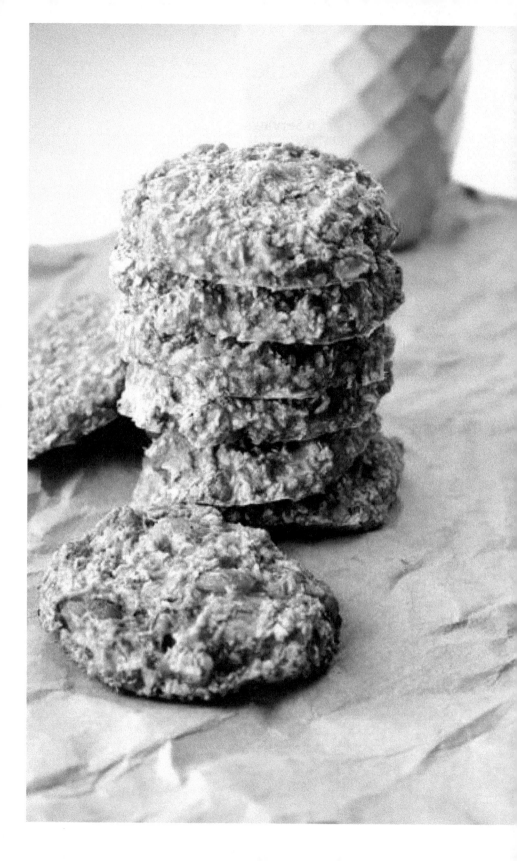

Dates Rice

6 Servings

Preparation Time: 30 minutes

Ingredients

- 6 Dates, chopped
- 1 cup Brown rice
- 2 cups Almond milk
- 2 tablespoons Cinnamon powder
- 2 tablespoons Coconut sugar

Directions

- In a pot, combine the rice with the milk and the other ingredients, bring to a simmer and cook over medium heat for 20 minutes.
- Stir the mix again, divide into bowls and serve for breakfast.

Coconut Porridge

6 Servings

Preparation Time: 30 minutes

Ingredients

- 1 cup Strawberries, halved
- 4 cups Coconut milk
- 1 cup Cornmeal
- 1 teaspoon Vanilla extract
- ½ teaspoon Nutmeg, ground

Directions

- Put the milk in a pot, bring to a simmer over medium heat, add the cornmeal and the other ingredients, toss, cook for 20 minutes, and take off the heat.
- Divide the porridge between plates and serve for breakfast.

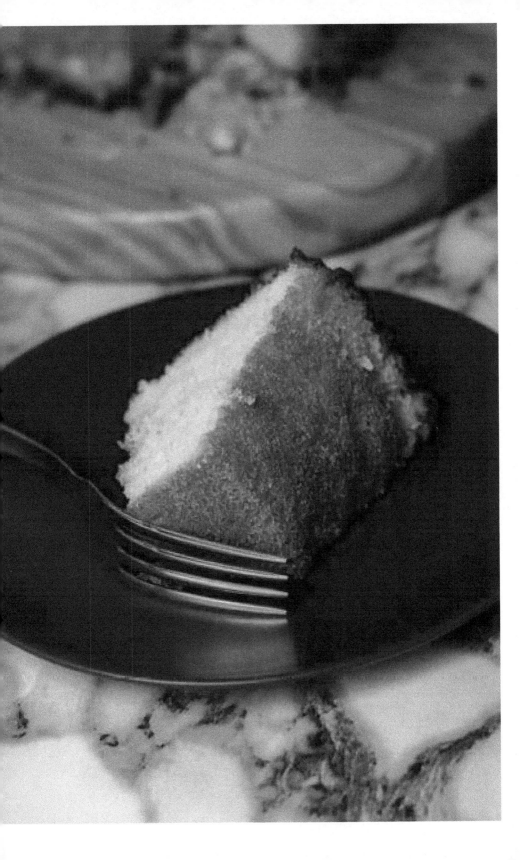

Berries Rice

6 Servings

Preparation Time: 30 minutes

Ingredients

- 1 tablespoon Cinnamon powder
- 1 cup Brown rice
- 2 cups Coconut milk
- 1 cup Blackberries
- ½ cup Coconut cream, unsweetened

Directions

- Put the milk in a pot, bring to a simmer over medium heat, add the rice and the other ingredients, cook for 20 minutes, and divide into bowls.
- Serve warm for breakfast.

JUICES & SMOOTHIES

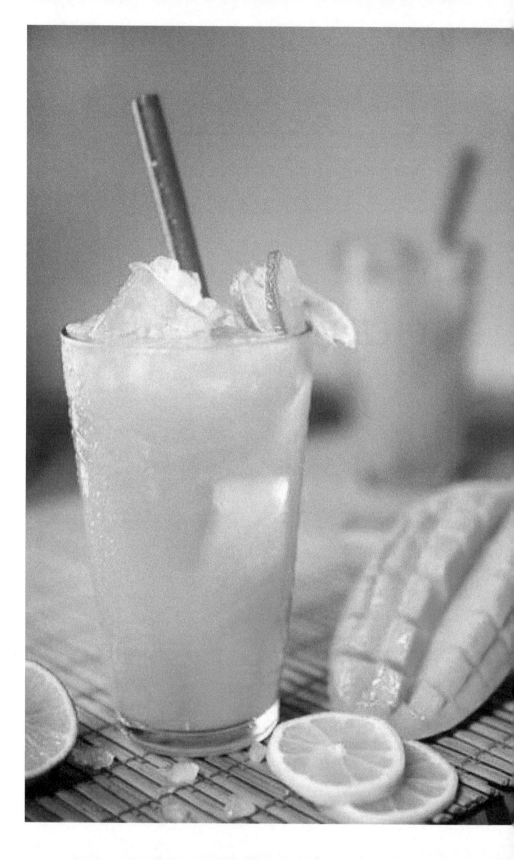

Carrot Juice

2 Servings

Preparation Time: 7 minutes

Ingredients

- 8 large Carrots, peeled and chopped
- Pinch of Ground Black pepper

Directions

- In a food processor, add carrot pieces and extract the juice according to the manufacturer's directions.
- Transfer into 2 glasses and stir in Black pepper. Serve immediately.

Red Fruit & Veggies Juice

3 Servings

Preparation Time: 12 minutes

Ingredients

- 3 medium red Beets, trimmed, peeled and chopped
- 2½ C. fresh Strawberries, hulled
- 2 large red Bell pepper, seeded and chopped
- 2 large Tomato, seeded and chopped
- ¼ C. fresh Mint leaves

Directions

- In a food processor, add all ingredients and extract the juice according to the manufacturer's directions.
- Transfer into 3 glasses and serve immediately.

Green Fruit & Veggie Juice

4 Servings

Preparation Time: 15 minutes

Ingredients

- 4 small green Apples, cored and sliced
- 4 C. fresh Spinach leaves
- 2Lemon, peeled and seeded
- 4 small Pears, cored and sliced
- 8 medium Celery stalks, chopped

Directions

- In a food processor, add all ingredients and extract the juice according to the manufacturer's directions.
- Transfer into 4 glasses and serve immediately.

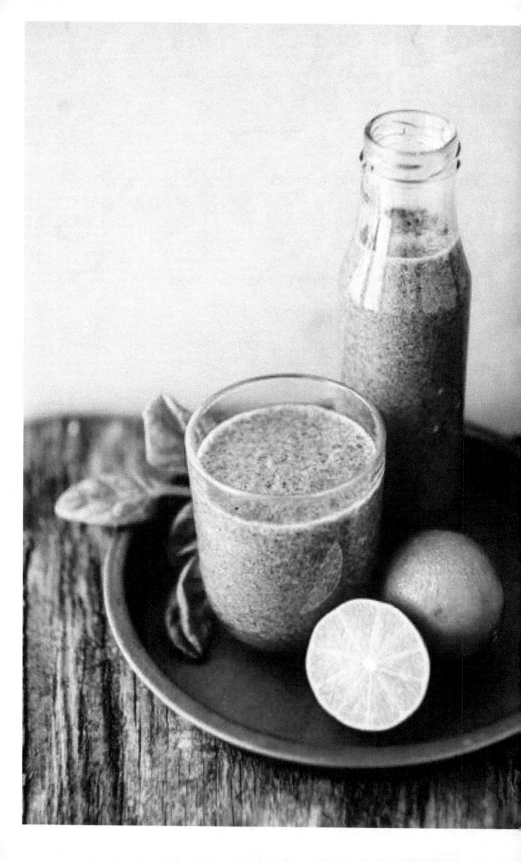

Mixed Veggie Juice

4 Servings

Preparation Time: 15 minutes

Ingredients

- 6 C. fresh Spinach
- 4 large seedless Cucumbers, peeled and chopped
- Pinch of ground Black pepper
- 4 medium fresh Tomatoes, chopped
- 5 large Celery stalks, chopped
- 5 tbsps fresh Basil leaves

Directions

- In a food processor, add all ingredients and extract the juice according to the manufacturer's directions.
- Transfer into 4 glasses and serve immediately.

Oat & Orange Smoothie

4 Servings

Preparation Time: 12 minutes

Ingredients

- 2/3 C. rolled Oats

- 2 large frozen Bananas, peeled and sliced
- 1 C. Ice cubes
- 2 large Oranges, peeled, seeded and sectioned
- 2½ C. unsweetened Almond Milk

Directions

- In a high-speed blender, add rolled Oats and pulse until finely chopped.
- Add remaining all ingredients and pulse until smooth.
- Transfer into 4 serving glasses and serve immediately.

Mango Smoothie

3 Servings

Preparation Time: 12 minutes

Ingredients

- 2 medium Mangoes, peeled, pitted and chopped
- ½ tsp. Organic Vanilla extract
- 1 medium Bananas, peeled and sliced
- 2 tbsps Almonds, chopped
- 1½ C. chilled fat-free Milk

Directions

- In a high-speed blender, add all ingredients and pulse until smooth.
- Transfer into 3 serving glasses and serve immediately.

Blueberry Smoothie

4 Servings

Preparation Time: 15 minutes

Ingredients

- 2 C. frozen Blueberries
- 1 C. unsweetened Almond Milk
- 1 small Banana, peeled and sliced
- ¼ C. Ice cubes

Directions

- In a high-speed blender, add all ingredients and pulse until smooth.
- Transfer into 4 serving glasses and serve immediately.

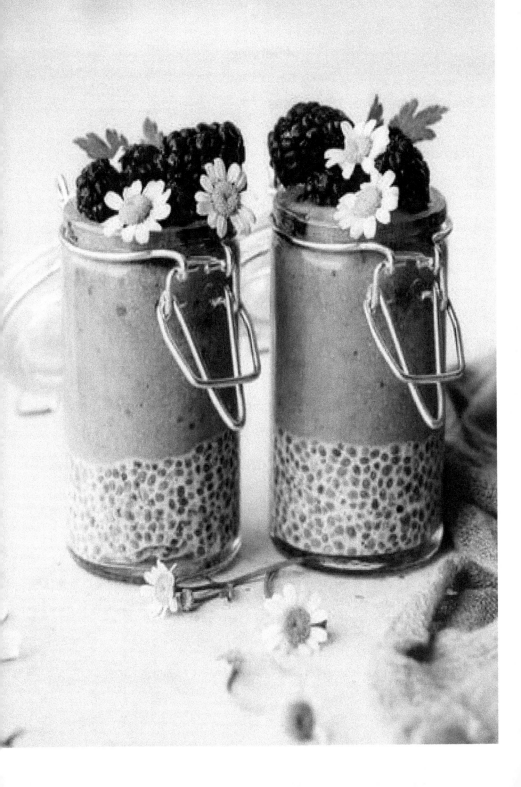

Strawberry Smoothie

4 Servings

Preparation Time: 15 minutes

Ingredients

- 1 C. fresh Strawberries, hulled and sliced
- 1½ C. chilled fat-free Milk
- 1 frozen large Banana, peeled and sliced
- 2 tbsps unsalted Almonds

Directions

- In a high-speed blender, add all ingredients and pulse until smooth.
- Transfer into 4 serving glasses and serve immediately.

LUNCH

Garlicky Shrimp

2 Servings

Preparation Time: 15 minutes

Ingredients

- 1 tbsp Olive Oil
- 1 Serrano pepper, seeded and chopped finely
- 1 tsp. fresh lemon juice
- 2 Garlic cloves, minced
- ½ lb. shrimp, peeled and deveined
- 1 tbsp fresh Cilantro, chopped

Directions

- In a large pan, heat the oil over medium heat and sauté Garlic and Serrano pepper for about 1 minute.
- Add shrimp and cook for about 4-5 minutes or until done completely.
- Stir in lemon juice and remove from heat. Serve hot with the topping of Cilantro.

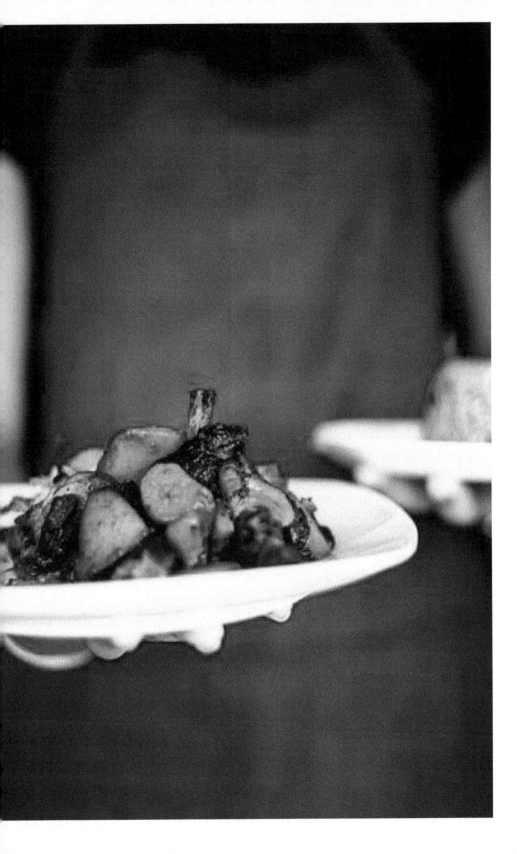

Shrimp with Asparagus

4 Servings

Preparation Time: 25 minutes

Ingredients

- 2 tbsps Olive Oil

- 1 lb. shrimp, peeled and deveined

- 2 tbsps fresh lemon juice

- 1 lb. asparagus, trimmed

- 4 Garlic cloves, minced

- 1/3 C. low-sodium chicken broth

Directions

- In a large pan, heat the oil over medium-high heat. Add all the ingredients except for broth and cook for about 2 minutes, without stirring.

- Stir the mixture and cook for about 3-4 minutes, stirring occasionally. Stir in the broth and cook for about 2-4 more minutes.

- Serve hot.

Shrimp with Kale

4 Servings

Preparation Time: 25 minutes

Ingredients

- 1 lb. medium shrimp, peeled and deveined
- 4 Garlic cloves, chopped finely
- 1 lb. fresh kale, tough ribs removed and chopped
- 1 medium Onion, chopped
- 1 fresh red chili, sliced
- ¼ C. low-sodium chicken broth

Directions

- In a large non-stick pan, heat 1 tbsp of the oil over medium-high heat and cook the shrimp for about 2 minutes per side. With a slotted spoon,
- Transfer the shrimp onto a plate. In the same pan, heat the remaining 2 tbsps of oil over medium heat and sauté the Garlic and red chili for about 1 minute.

- Add the kale and broth and cook for about 4-5 minutes, stirring occasionally. Stir in the cooked shrimp and cook for about 1 minute. Serve hot.

Beef & Veggie Meatloaf

8 Servings

Preparation Time: 60 minutes

Ingredients

- 2 lbs. lean ground Beef
- ½ C. Green Bell Pepper, seeded and chopped
- 2 Garlic cloves, minced
- ½ C. salt-free ketchup
- Freshly ground Black pepper, to taste
- ½ C. Onion, chopped
- 1 C. low-fat cheddar cheese, grated
- 1 tsp. dried thyme, crushed
- 3 C. fresh spinach, chopped
- 1½ C. part-skim mozzarella cheese, grated

Directions

- Preheat the oven to 350 °F. Lightly. Grease a baking dish. In a large bowl, add all ingredients except for spinach and mozzarella cheese and mix until well combined. Place a large wax paper onto a smooth surface.

- Place meat mixture over wax paper. Place spinach over meat mixture, pressing slightly. Top with mozzarella cheese evenly. Roll the wax paper around meat mixture to form a meatloaf. Carefully remove the wax paper and place the meatloaf onto prepared baking dish.
- Bake for about 1-1¼ hours. Remove from oven and set aside for about 10 minutes before serving. With a sharp knife cut into desired sized slices and serve.

Beef & Veggies Chili

8 Servings

Preparation Time: 3 hours 10 minutes

Ingredients

- 2 lbs. lean ground Beef
- ½ C. Green Bell Pepper, seeded and chopped
- 4 oz. fresh mushrooms, sliced
- 1 (6-oz.) can salt-free tomato paste
- 1 tbsp ground cumin
- Freshly ground Black pepper, to taste
- 1 yellow Onion, chopped
- ½ C. carrot, peeled and chopped
- 2 Garlic cloves, minced
- 2 tbsps red chili powder
- Pinch of salt
- 4 C. water

Directions

- Heat a large non-stick pan over medium-high heat and cook Beef for about 8-10 minutes. Drain the excess grease from pan. Stir in remaining ingredients and bring to a boil. Reduce the heat to low and cook, covered for about 3 hours. Serve hot.

Beef & Veggie Meatballs

4 Servings

Preparation Time: 30 minutes

Ingredients

- ¾ C. carrot, peeled and grated
- Pinch of salt
- 1 egg, beaten
- 1 Garlic clove, minced
- Freshly ground Black pepper, to taste
- ¾ C. zucchini, grated
- 1 lb. lean ground Beef
- ¼ of a small Onion, chopped finely
- 2 tbsps fresh Cilantro, chopped finely
- 6 C. fresh baby greens

Directions

- Preheat the oven to 400 °F. Line a large baking sheet with parchment paper. Set a large colander in the sink.

47

Add carrot and zucchini and sprinkle with 2 pinches of salt. Set aside for at least 10 minutes.

- Transfer the veggies over a paper towel and squeeze out all the moisture of veggies. In a large mixing bowl, add squeezed vegetables, Beef, egg, Onion, Garlic, Cilantro, salt and Black pepper and mix until well combined.

- Shape the mixture into equal-sized balls. Arrange the meatballs onto the prepared baking sheet in a single layer. Bake for about 25-30 minutes or until done completely. Serve these meatballs with fresh greens.

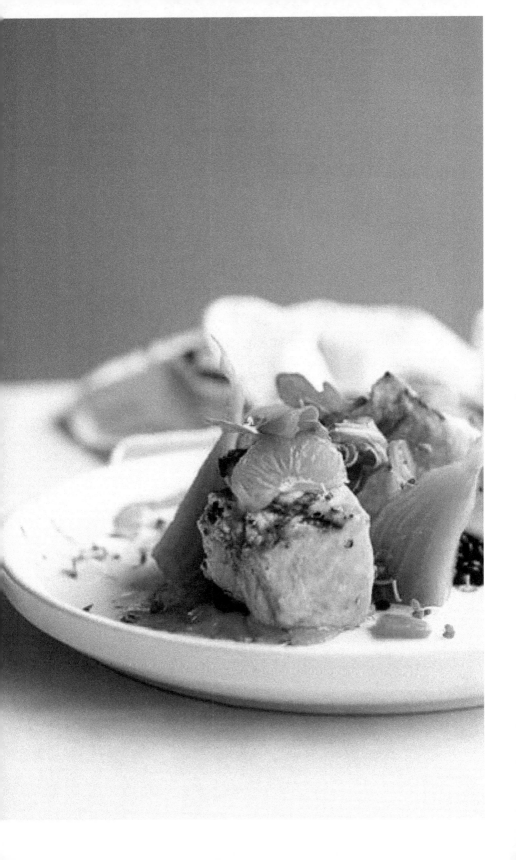

Chicken with spinach

4 Servings

Preparation Time: 25 minutes

Ingredients

- 2 tbsps unsalted margarine, divided
- 2 Garlic cloves, minced
- ¼ C. low-fat Parmesan cheese, shredded
- Freshly ground Black pepper, to taste
- 1 lb. skinless, boneless Chicken tenders
- 10 oz. frozen chopped Spinach, thawed
- ¼ C. low-fat Sour cream

Directions

- In a large pan, melt 1 tbsp of margarine over medium-high heat and cook chicken for about 3-4 minutes from both sides.
- Transfer the chicken into a bowl. In the same pan, melt the remaining margarine over medium-low heat and

sauté Garlic for about 1 minute. Add spinach and cook for about 1 minute. Add cheese, cream and Black pepper and stir to combine. Spread the spinach mixture in the bottom of pan evenly.

- Place chicken over spinach in a single layer. Immediately, reduce the heat to low and simmer, covered for about 5 minutes or until desired doneness of chicken. Serve hot.

Chicken with zucchini

6 Servings

Preparation Time: 30 minutes

Ingredients

- 2 tbsps Olive Oil, divided
- Pinch of salt
- Freshly ground Black pepper, to taste
- 1½ lb. zucchini, sliced
- 1 tsp. fresh lemon zest, grated finely
- 1 lb. skinless, boneless chicken breasts, cut into bite-sized pieces
- 2 Garlic cloves, minced
- 2 tbsps fresh lemon juice
- 2 tbsps fresh parsley, minced

Directions

- In a large pan, heat 1 tbsp of oil over medium heat and stir fry chicken pieces for about 4-5 minutes or until golden brown from all sides.
- Transfer the chicken into a plate. In the same pan, heat the remaining oil over medium heat and sauté Garlic for about 1 minute. Add zucchini and cook for about 5-6 minutes. Stir in chicken and cook for about 2 minutes. Stir in lemon juice, zest and parsley and remove from heat. Serve warm.

Chicken with bell peppers

6 servings

Preparation Time: 35 minutes

Ingredients

- 3 tbsps Olive Oil, divided
- 1 medium Onion, sliced
- 1 tsp. dried oregano, crushed
- ¼ tsp. ground Cumin
- ¼ C. low-sodium Chicken broth
- 3 bell Peppers, seeded and sliced
- 1 lb. boneless, skinless Chicken breasts, sliced thinly
- Freshly ground Black pepper, to taste

Directions

- In a pan, heat 1 tbsp of oil over medium-high heat and cook the bell peppers and Onion slices for about 4-5 minutes.

- With a slotted spoon, transfer the peppers mixture onto a plate. In the same pan over medium-high heat and cook the chicken for about 8 minutes, stirring frequently. Stir in the thyme, spices, salt, Black pepper, and broth, and bring to a boil. Add the peppers mixture and stir to combine.
- Reduce the heat to medium and cook for about 3–5 minutes or until all the liquid is absorbed, stirring occasionally. Serve immediately.

SNACKS & SIDES

Basil Olives Mix

5 Servings

Preparation Time: 5minutes

Ingredients

- 2 tablespoons Olive oil
- 1 tablespoon Balsamic vinegar
- A pinch of Black pepper
- 4 cups Corn
- 2 cups Black Olives, pitted and halved
- 1 red Onion, chopped
- ½ cup cherry Tomatoes, halved
- 1 tablespoon Basil, chopped
- 1 tablespoon Jalapeno, chopped
- 2 cups romaine Lettuce, shredded

Directions

- In a large bowl, combine the corn with the Olives, lettuce and the other ingredients, toss well, divide between plates and serve as a side dish.

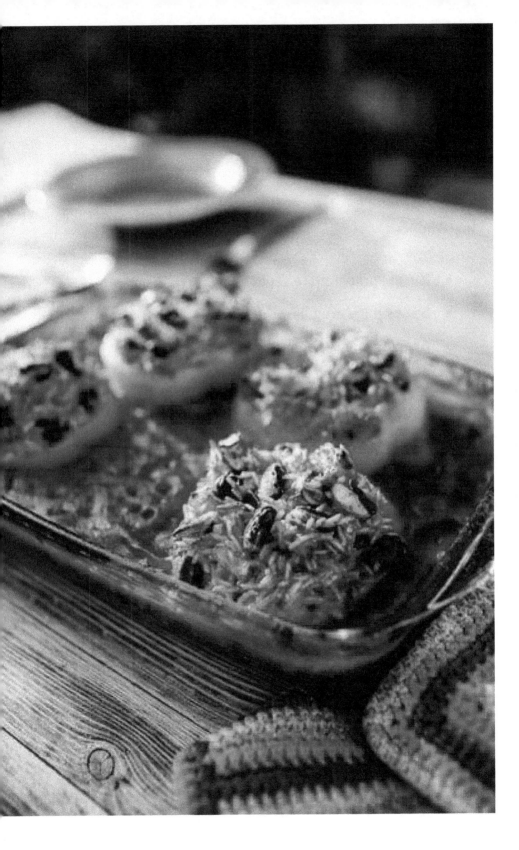

Arugula Salad

5 Servings

Preparation Time: 5 minutes

Ingredients

- ¼ cup Pomegranate seeds
- 5 cups Baby arugula
- 6 tablespoons green Onions, chopped
- 1 tablespoon Balsamic vinegar
- 2 tablespoons Olive oil
- 3 tablespoons Pine nuts
- ½ Shallot, chopped

Directions

- In a salad bowl, combine the arugula with the pomegranate and the other ingredients, toss and serve.

Green Beans Salad

5 Servings

Preparation Time: 5 minutes

Ingredients

- Juice of 1 Lime
- 2 cups romaine Lettuce, shredded
- 1 cup Corn
- ½ pound Green beans, blanched and halved
- 1 Cucumber, chopped
- 1/3 cup Chives, chopped

Directions

- In a bowl, combine the green beans with the corn and the other ingredients, toss and serve.

Chives Edamame Salad

5 Servings

Preparation Time: 10 minutes

Ingredients

- 2 tablespoons Olive oil
- 2 tablespoons Balsamic vinegar
- 2 Garlic cloves, minced
- 3 cups Edamame, shelled
- 1 tablespoon Chives, chopped
- 2 Shallots, chopped

Directions

- Heat up a pan with the oil over medium heat, add the edamame, the garlic and the other ingredients, toss, cook for 6 minutes, divide between plates and serve.

Grapes and Cucumber Salad

4 Servings

Preparation Time: 5 minutes

Ingredients

- 2 cups Baby spinach
- 2 Avocados, peeled, pitted and roughly cubed
- 1 Cucumber, sliced
- 1 and ½ cups Green grapes, halved
- 2 tablespoons Avocado oil
- 1 tablespoon Cider vinegar
- 2 tablespoons Parsley, chopped
- A pinch of Black pepper

Directions

- In a salad bowl, combine the baby spinach with the avocados and the other ingredients, toss and serve.

Parmesan Eggplant Mix

5 Servings

Preparation Time: 30 minutes

Ingredients

- 2 big Eggplants, roughly cubed
- 1 tablespoon Oregano, chopped
- ½ cup low-fat Parmesan, grated
- ¼ teaspoon Garlic powder
- 2 tablespoons Olive oil
- A pinch of Black pepper

Directions

- In a baking pan combine the eggplants with the oregano and the other ingredients except the cheese and toss.
- Sprinkle parmesan on top, introduce in the oven and bake at 370 degrees F for 20 minutes.
- Divide between plates and serve as a side dish.

Garlic Tomatoes Mix

4 Servings

Preparation Time: 30 minutes

Ingredients

- 2 pounds Tomatoes, halved
- 1 tablespoon Basil, chopped
- 3 tablespoons Olive oil
- Zest of 1 Lemon, grated
- 3 Garlic cloves, minced
- ¼ cup low-fat Parmesan, grated
- A pinch of Black pepper

Directions

- In a baking pan, combine the tomatoes with the basil and the other ingredients except the cheese and toss.
- Sprinkle the parmesan on top, introduce in the oven at 375 degrees F for 20 minutes, divide between plates and serve as a side dish.

Parsley Mushrooms

5 Servings

Preparation Time: 40minutes

Ingredients

- 2 pounds white Mushrooms, halved
- 4 Garlic cloves, minced
- 2 tablespoons Olive oil
- 1 tablespoon Thyme, chopped
- 2 tablespoons Parsley, chopped
- Black pepper to the taste

Directions

- In a baking pan, combine the mushrooms with the garlic and the other ingredients, toss, introduce in the oven and cook at 400 degrees F for 30 minutes.
- Divide between plates and serve as a side dish.

DINNER

Chickpeas Stew

4 Servings

Preparation Time: 30 minutes

Ingredients

- 1 tablespoon Olive Oil

- 1 yellow Onion, chopped

- 2 teaspoons chili powder

- 14 ounces Canned chickpeas, no-salt-added, drained and rinsed

- 14 ounces Canned tomatoes, no-salt-added, cubed

- 1 cup low-sodium chicken stock

- 1 tablespoon Cilantro, chopped

- A pinch of Black pepper

Directions

- Heat up a pot with the oil over medium-high heat, add the Onion and chili powder, stir and cook for 5 minutes.

- Add the chickpeas and the other ingredients, toss, cook for 15 minutes over medium heat, divide into bowls and serve for lunch.

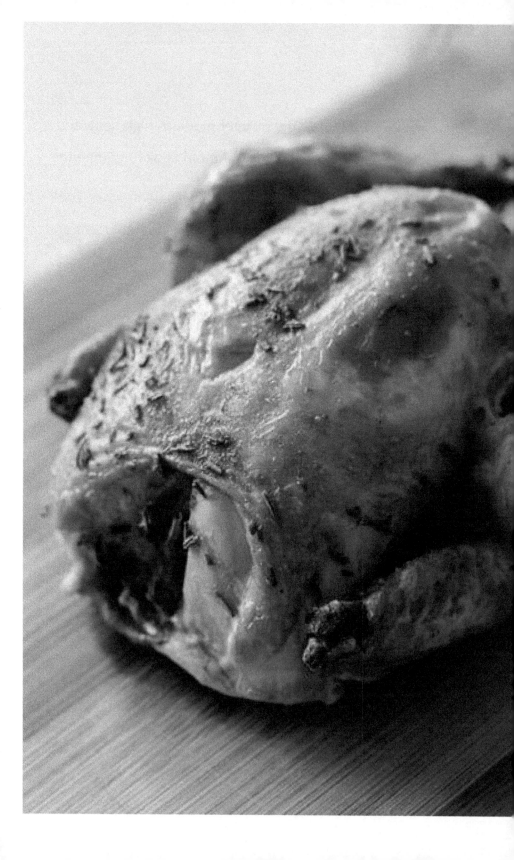

Lemon Chicken Salad

4 Servings

Preparation Time: 10 minutes

Ingredients

- 1 tablespoon Olive Oil
- A pinch of Black pepper
- 2 rotisserie chicken, skinless, boneless, shredded
- 1 pound cherry tomatoes, halved
- 1 red Onion, chopped
- 4 cups baby spinach
- ¼ cup walnuts, chopped
- ½ teaspoon lemon zest, grated
- 2 tablespoons lemon juice

Directions

- In a salad bowl, combine the chicken with the tomato and the other ingredients, toss and serve for lunch.

Asparagus Salad

Preparation Time: 30 minutes

Ingredients

- 3 Garlic cloves, minced
- 2 tablespoons Olive Oil
- 1 red Onion, chopped
- 3 carrots, sliced
- ½ cup low-sodium chicken stock
- 2 cups baby spinach
- 1 pound asparagus, trimmed and halved
- 1 red bell pepper, cut into strips
- 1 yellow bell pepper, cut into strips
- 1 Green Bell Pepper, cut into strips
- A pinch of Black pepper

Directions

- Heat up a pan with the oil over medium-high heat, add the Onion and the Garlic, stir and sauté for 2 minutes.
- Add the asparagus and the other ingredients except the spinach, toss, and cook for 15 minutes.
- Add the spinach, cook everything for 3 minutes more, divide into bowls and serve for lunch.

Rosemary Pork Chops

4 Servings

Preparation Time: 25 minutes

Ingredients

- 4 pork chops
- 1 tablespoon Olive Oil
- 2 shallots, chopped
- 1 pound white mushrooms, sliced
- ½ cup low-sodium Beef stock
- 1 tablespoon rosemary, chopped
- ¼ teaspoon Garlic powder
- 1 teaspoon sweet paprika

Directions

- Heat up a pan with the oil over medium-high heat, add the pork chops and the shallots, toss brown for 10 minutes and transfer to a slow cooker.

- Add the rest of the ingredients, put the lid on and cook on Low for 8 hours.
- Divide the pork chops and mushrooms between plates and serve for lunch.

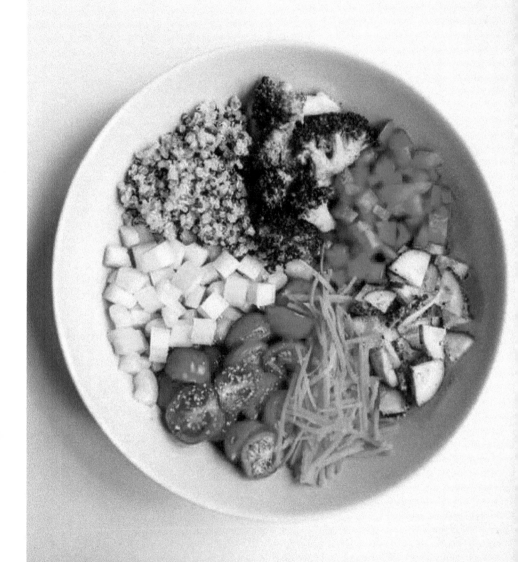

Eggplant and Tomato Stew

4 Servings

Preparation Time: 25 minutes

Ingredients

- 1 pound Eggplants, roughly cubed

- 2 Garlic cloves, minced

- 2 tablespoons Olive Oil

- 1 yellow Onion, chopped

- 1 teaspoon Sweet paprika

- ½ cup Cilantro, chopped

- 14 ounces low-sodium Canned tomatoes, chopped

- 1 tablespoon Cilantro, chopped

Directions

- Heat up a pan with the oil over medium-high heat; add the Onion and the Garlic and sauté for 2 minutes.

- Add the eggplant and the other ingredients except the Cilantro bring to a simmer and cook for 18 minutes.

- Divide into bowls and serve with the Cilantro sprinkled on top.

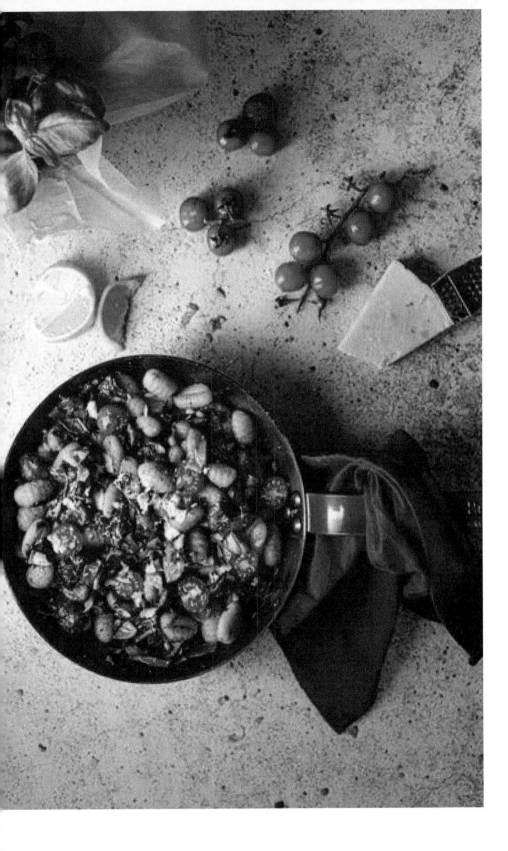

Beef and Scallions Mix

4 Servings

Preparation Time: 40 minutes

Ingredients

- 1 pound Beef stew meat, cubed
- 1 cup Canned tomatoes, no-salt-added and chopped
- 1 cup Scallions, chopped
- ¼ cup Parsley, chopped
- 1 and ¼ cups low-sodium Beef stock
- 1 yellow Onion, chopped
- 1 tablespoon Olive Oil
- 2 cups Peas
- Black Pepper to the taste

Directions

- Heat up a pot with the oil over medium-high heat, add the Onion and the meat and brown for 5 minutes.

- Add the peas and the other ingredients stir bring to a simmer and cook over medium heat for 25 minutes more.
- Divide the mix into bowls and serve for lunch.

Lime Turkey Stew

4 Servings

Preparation Time: 35 minutes

Ingredients

- 2 tablespoons Olive Oil
- 1 Turkey breast, skinless, boneless and cubed
- 1 cup low-sodium Beef stock
- 1 cup Tomato puree, low sodium
- ¼ teaspoon Lime zest, grated
- 1 yellow Onion, chopped
- 1 tablespoon Sweet paprika
- 1 tablespoon Cilantro, chopped
- 2 tablespoons Lime juice
- ¼ teaspoon Ginger, grated

Directions

- Heat up a pot with the oil over medium-high heat, add the Onion and the meat and brown for 5 minutes.

- Add the stock and the other ingredients bring to a simmer and cook over medium heat for 25 minutes.
- Divide the mix into bowls and serve for lunch.

Beef and Beans Salad

4 Servings

Preparation Time: 30 minutes

Ingredients

- 1 pound Beef stew meat, cut into strips
- 1 tablespoon sage, chopped
- 1 tablespoon Olive Oil
- A pinch of Black pepper
- ½ teaspoon Cumin, ground
- 2 cups Cherry tomatoes, cubed
- 1 Avocado, peeled, pitted and cubed
- 1 cup Canned Black Beans, , no-salt-added, drained and rinsed
- ½ cup Green Onions, chopped
- 2 tablespoons Lime juice
- 2 tablespoons Balsamic vinegar
- 2 tablespoons Cilantro, chopped

Directions

- Heat up a pan with the oil over medium-high heat, add the meat and brown for 5 minutes.
- Add the sage, Black pepper and the cumin, toss and cook for 5 minutes more.
- Add the rest of the ingredients, toss, reduce heat to medium and cook the mix for 20 minutes.
- Divide the salad into bowls and serve for lunch.

Squash and Peppers Stew

4 Servings

Preparation Time: 30 minutes

Ingredients

- 1 pound Squash, peeled and roughly cubed

- 1 cup low-sodium chicken stock

- 1 cup Canned tomatoes, no-salt-added, crushed

- 1 tablespoon Olive Oil

- 1 red Onion, chopped

- 2 orange Sweet peppers, chopped

- ½ cup Quinoa

- ½ tablespoon Chives, chopped

Directions

- Heat up a pot with the oil over medium heat; add the Onion, stir and sauté for 2 minutes.

- Add the squash and the other ingredients bring to a simmer, and cook for 15 minutes.

- Stir the stew, divide into bowls and serve for lunch.

DESSERTS

Mixed Fruit Bowl

8 Servings

Preparation Time: 15 minutes

Ingredients

- ½ C. fresh Strawberries, hulled and sliced
- 1 C. Banana, peeled and sliced
- ½ C. fresh Blueberries
- 2 tbsps Maple syrup
- 2 tbsps Almonds, chopped
- ½ C. fresh Cherries, pitted and halved
- 1 tbsp fresh Lemon juice

Directions

- In a large bowl, add fruit, maple syrup and lemon juice and gently toss to coat well. Place fruit mixture into serving bowls. Top with almonds and serve.

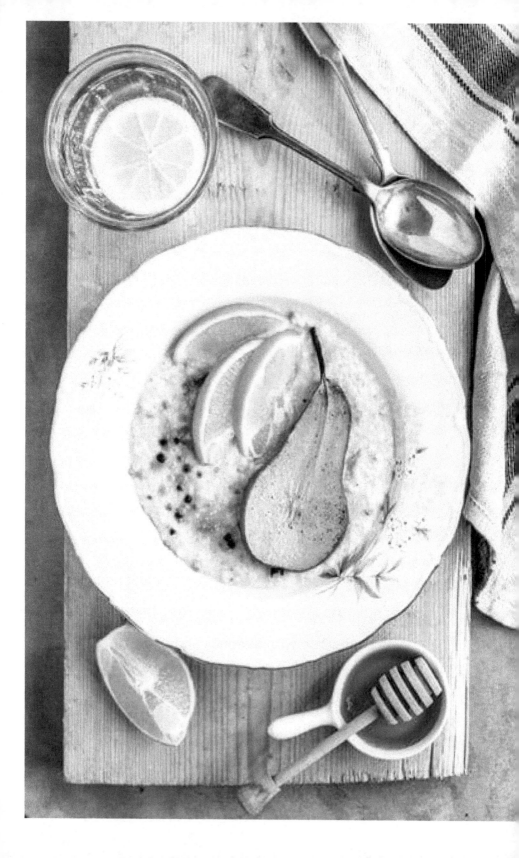

Stuffed Apples

6 Servings

Preparation Time: 50 minutes

Ingredients

- 1 tsp. Ground cinnamon
- ¾ C. Oats
- 3 tbsps unsweetened Applesauce
- ¼ tsp. ground Ginger
- 6 large Apples
- ¾ C. Pecans, chopped
- 1/8 tsp. Ground allspice
- ¾ C. Water

Directions

- Preheat the oven to 350 °F. In a bowl, mix together the oats, pecans, applesauce and spices. Set aside.
- Remove the top of each apple. With a spoon, carefully scoop out the flesh from inside of the apples.

- Stuff the apples with pecan mixture evenly. Arrange the apples into a baking dish.

- Add water in the baking dish. Bake for about 30-40 minutes. Serve warm.

Frozen Avocado Yogurt

6 Servings

Preparation Time: 10 minutes

Ingredients

- ½ C. fat-free plain Greek Yogurt
- 2 medium Avocados, peeled, pitted and chopped
- 3 tbsps powdered Stevia
- 1 tsp. organic Vanilla extract
- ½ C. unsweetened Almond milk
- 1 tbsp fresh Lemon juice
- 1 tsp. fresh Mint leaves

Directions

- In a blender, add all ingredients except mint leaves and pulse until creamy and smooth.
- Transfer into an airtight container and freeze for at least 2-3 hours.

- Remove from freezer and set aside in room temperature for about 10-15 minutes.
- With a spoon, stir well. Top with fresh mint leaves and serve.

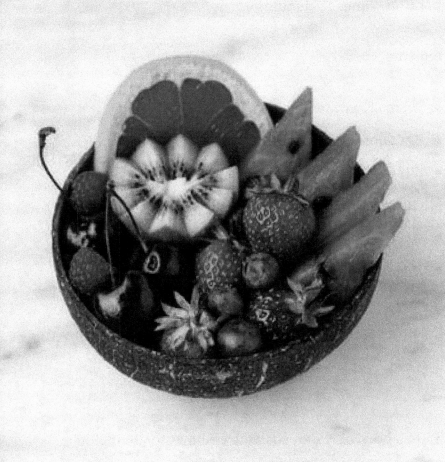

Raspberry Ice Cream

8 Servings

Preparation Time: 15 minutes

Ingredients

- 1 small Avocado, peeled, pitted and chopped
- ¼ C. unsalted Cashews
- 2¼ C. fresh Raspberries, divided
- 10 Dates, pitted and chopped
- 1¾ C. unsweetened Almond milk
- 1 tbsp fresh Lemon juice
- 2/3 C. filtered Water
- 1 tbsp fresh Beet juice

Directions

- In a bowl of water, soak the cashews for 30 minutes. Drain the cashews well.
- In a blender, add 2 C. of raspberries and reaming all ingredients and pulse until creamy and smooth.

- Transfer into an ice cream maker and process according to manufacturer's directions.

- Transfer into an airtight container and freeze for at least 4-5 hours. Top with the remaining raspberries and serve.

Pumpkin Ice Cream

8 Servings

Preparation Time: 10 minutes

Ingredients

- ½ C. Dates, pitted and chopped

- 15 oz. homemade Pumpkin puree

- 2 (14-oz.) cans unsweetened Coconut milk

- 1½ tsps. . Pumpkin pie spice

- ½ tsp. organic Vanilla extract

- ½ tsp. ground Cinnamon

Directions

- In a high-speed blender, add all the ingredients and pulse until smooth.

- Transfer into an airtight container and freeze for about 1-2 hours.

- Now, transfer the mixture into an ice cream maker and process it according to the manufacturer's directions.

- Return the ice cream to the airtight container and freeze for about 1-2 hours before serving.

Peach Sorbet

8 Servings

Preparation Time: 10 minutes

Ingredients

- 1¾ C. unsweetened Coconut milk

- 6 medium Peaches, pitted and chopped

- 1 tsp. organic Vanilla extract

- 3 tbsps unsalted Almonds, chopped

- ¼ tsp. ground Cinnamon

Directions

- In a blender, add peaches and pulse until a puree forms.

- Add remaining ingredients and pulse until smooth and creamy.

- Transfer the peach mixture into an ice-cream maker and process according to manufacturer's directions.

- Now, transfer into an airtight container and freeze for 4-5 hours or until set completely. Top with almonds and serve.

Spinach Sorbet

6 Servings

Preparation Time: 10 minutes

Ingredients

- 1 tbsp fresh Basil leaves

- ¾ C. Almond milk

- 3 C. fresh Spinach, torn

- ½ of Avocado, peeled, pitted and chopped

- 20 drops Liquid stevia

- 1 tsp. organic Vanilla extract

- 1 tsp. unsalted Almonds, chopped finely

- 1 C. Ice cubes

Directions

- In a blender, add all the ingredients and pulse until creamy and smooth.

- Transfer into an ice cream maker and process according to manufacturer's directions.

- Transfer into an airtight container and freeze for at least 4-5 hours before serving.

Berries Granita

6 Servings

Preparation Time: 10 minutes

Ingredients

- ½ C. fresh Raspberries

- ½ C. fresh Strawberries, hulled and sliced

- ½ C. fresh Blueberries

- 1 tbsp Maple syrup

- 1 C. Ice cubes, crushed

- ½ C. fresh Blackberries

- 1 tbsp fresh Lemon juice

Directions

- In a high-speed blender, add the berries, maple syrup, lemon juice, and ice cubes and pulse on high speed until smooth.

- Transfer the berry mixture into an 8x8-inch baking dish, spread evenly, and freeze for at least 30 minutes.

- Remove from the freezer and, with a fork, stir the granita completely. Freeze for 2-3 hours, stirring every 30 minutes with a fork.

Lightning Source UK Ltd.
Milton Keynes UK
UKHW020703310521
384670UK00006B/134